From the Author

Ok, let's be honest. Kids wake up in the morning and the last thing they want to do is SIT AROUND IN CLASS or BE CALM.

They want to RELEASE SOME ENERGY!

With this book, you can choose a variety of quick and simple moves that EXERCISE THE BODY AND THE BRAIN!

Ideally used in a classroom or at your home, pick an activity or two and help get those morning, afternoon, or evening wigglies out!

Let's give these kids what they want... MOVEMENT!

Exercise the mind and body with the newest addition to the Super Smart Science Series!

Use your imagination and create your own activities on the last 5 pages!

-April Chloe Terrazas

for HOME or CLASS

Super Smart Workout Series

Sweet moves and activities by:

April Chloe Terrazas

Super Smart Workout Series. ISBN: 978-0-9843848-6-0. April Chloe Terrazas, BS University of Texas at Austin.
Copyright © 2013 Crazy Brainz, LLC

Visit us on the web! **www.Crazy-Brainz.com**

This book is Dedicated To:

All kids who want to *have fun* and *move around* at home and in the classroom!

AND to the *AWESOME* *Parents* and *Teachers* who use this book and make their families and classes *happy* and *productive*!

*Always participate in the following activities under adult supervision.

Table oF Contents

24. Crazy stretch
25. Dance party
26. Shake it like a happy kid
27. Count to 20
28. free moves!
29. Airplane
30. Soccer Star
31. Pick the fruit tree!
32. Marching Band
33. Twist and smile
34. Pick a strawberry, pick an apple
35. Popcorn!
36. Sway Like a Tree
37. Toss The Ball
38. Foot-Alphabet
39. Arm -Alphabet
40. Flap like a bird

Jump Around!

Jump around from side to side and as high as you possibly can!

While jumping, say the following words:

Science

Biology

Physics

Chemistry

(or choose 4 spelling words to repeat)

Options:
Jump for 30 seconds
Jump for 60 seconds
Jump for 90 seconds

Count it

Pick one of the following numbers and count backwards to zero while jogging in place!

24	13	9	18
51	27	36	46
39	42	27	32
17	33	25	55

(or choose your own number!)

Dolphin Fun-dip

Do the Dolphin Fun-Dip!

What does a dolphin do?
It jumps in and out of the water!
**Dip your body down
and jump up like a dolphin!**

*While jumping, take turns naming
things that live in the ocean.*
For example: Fish, Crab, Shark, Coral

Options:
Dolphin Fun-Dip for 60 seconds
Dolphin Fun-Dip for 2 minutes

Spell it #1

Pick one of the following words and <u>spell it out loud while marching in place!</u>

(Then repeat with another word)

Basketball	Author	Fearless
Playground	Tomorrow	Brave
People	Governor	Clothing

(Or choose your own spelling words)

Count to 30

Count to 30 while doing...

Options:

Jumping Jacks

Side bends

Running in place

Dancing in place

(Repeat)

Stretch Like A Cat

Have you ever seen a cat stretch?

They bend and move their bodies in all different directions!

Bend and move and stretch your body like a cat!

While stretching, count in multiples of:

2   4   6

8   10   5

20   50   100

Ski Down The Mountain

JUMP FROM SIDE TO SIDE
like a professional skier coming down the mountain!

Swish! Swish! Swish!

**While you are skiing,
choose from the following options:**

-Name animals that live in the mountains
-Name clothes you would wear to ski
-Practice times tables
(with a partner or teacher)

Spell it #2

Pick one of the following words and <u>spell it out loud while rotating your arms in big circles!</u>

(Then repeat with another word)

Unusual	Toothbrush	Cream
Apple	Today	Create
Another	Teacher	Intelligent

(Or choose your own spelling words)

Run like a wild child!

Run in place like a WILD CHILD!

Move your arms around and bring your knees as high as you can while running in place.

While you are running,
choose from the following options:

-Count by 5's to 100

-Name as many animals that you can

-Name fruits and vegetables

How Many?

How many people are in the room?

Jump up as high as you can and reach for the sky that many times.

For example, if there are 15 people in the room, jump up and reach for the sky 15 times!

OR

Count to that number while doing jumping jacks.

For example, if there are 20 people in the room, do 20 jumping jacks!

Count to TEN

Practice counting to 10 in ENGLISH, then in SPANISH!

Uno   Dos   Tres   Cuatro

Cinco   Seis   Siete   Ocho

Nueve   Diez

While you are counting,
squat down with your knees bent and step side to side.

AROUND
the table

Side-step quickly around your desk or a nearby table while...

OPTIONS:

-Counting by 2's to 50

-Name as many vegetables as you can

-Name all the colors you can see

Reach for the stars!

Imagine you are looking at the night sky and you are going to jump up and reach for a star!

While you are jumping:

Name the planets in the Solar System

OR

Jump until you have gotten 20 stars!

tour of the land

Walk around the edge
(or perimeter)
of the room you are in right now.
As you are walking, practice your TIMES TABLES.

Choose one of the following numbers
and review times 1 through 10.
Then move to another number and repeat.

2   3   4   5   6

7   8   9   10

Spell it #3

Pick one of the following words and spell it out loud while standing and bringing your knees up high to your waist level.

Vocabulary from Book One of the Super Smart Science Series
Cellular Biology: Organelles, Structure, Function

Cell   Membrane   Cytoplasm

Mitochondria   Biology   Golgi

Centriole   Lysosome   Protein

(Or choose your own spelling words)

What Did They Say?

This is played with your teacher or parents and some friends!

Everyone listen to the grown-up and copy their movements WHILE answering their questions!

For example:

Grown-up: Move your arms and ask "What is 3x3?"

Kid: Imitate the movement and answer the question.

Count To 40

Count to 40
WHILE...

Option 1: **Hopping on one leg**

Option 2: **Doing jumping jacks**

Option 3: **Dancing**

Option 4: **Twisting from side to side**

Option 5: **Standing up tall and reaching for the sky, then bring your arms back to your side. (Repeat)**

Then repeat another option!

Count Your Toes

(This is a slower movement)

Standing up straight and tall, reach over and touch one toe (or the top of your shoe where that toe is) and say "1"!

Then stand up slowly to be straight and tall again and reach down for the next toe and say "2"!

Repeat for each toe until you have counted all 10 toes.

Crazy Stretch

Standing up straight and tall, reach over TO THE LEFT, then reach over TO THE RIGHT. Then reach down to the ground, and come back up standing tall.

Move your body in all different directions and stretch out your muscles!

While you are stretching:

1. Name as many cities in the United States as you can.

2. Count to 20, 30, 40, or 50

Dance party

While staying in your area, DANCE, DANCE, DANCE!

Move your arms and your legs
and have fun!

While you are dancing:

1. Play music to dance and sing with

2. Create your own song to dance to

3. Go around the room and everyone say what their favorite song is

4. Count by 5's to 50

Shake it like a happy kid!

**Dance your little heart out!
Move your body and have fun!**

Options:

Jump

Shake

Dance

Hop

Sway

Slide

Count to 20

Count to 20
WHILE...

Option 1: Hopping back and forth from one leg to another

Option 2: Squat down and jump straight up as high as possible!

Option 3: Rotating your arms in big circles

Option 4: Doing jumping jacks

Then repeat another option!

free moves!

<u>While staying in your area</u>, you are free to move around, stretch, jump, dance, hop, sway, and shake!

Jump to the sky!
Reach for your toes!
Bend to the left!
Bend to the right!
Dance!
Have fun!

(30 seconds, 1 minute or 2 minutes)

Airplane

Stand up straight and tall and move your arms and upper body around like an airplane flying through the sky!

While you are moving your arms and upper body,

1. Name the planets
2. Practice times tables
3. List vegetables
4. List fruits

Soccer Star

Stand up straight and tall and jump from left foot to right foot while bringing your knees high, just like a soccer star!

While you are jumping from left foot to right foot,
1. Count multiples of 2
2. Count multiples of 5
3. Count multiples of 10
4. Count multiples of 50

(30 seconds, 1 minute or 2 minutes)

Pick the fruit tree!

Stand up straight and tall and reach your arms up high, first your left arm then your right arm.

Go back and forth from left arm to right arm, picking from the fruit tree!

While you are picking fruit,
1. Count from 1 to 20
2. Count from 1 to 30
3. Count from 1 to 40
4. Count from 1 to 50

Marching Band

Pick one of the following numbers and count backwards to zero **while marching in place!**

25   33   12   21

45   17   56   57

34   22   26   24

19   63   35   15

(or choose your own number!)

Twist and smile

**Stand in place and twist your body!
Stand on your left leg and twist,
then stand on your right leg and twist.**

**Move your body in all
different directions and twist!**

While you are twisting and smiling:

1. Name cities in your home state

2. Count to 20, 30, 40, or 50

Pick a Strawberry, Pick an Apple!

Stand up straight and tall, reach over to your toes and pick a strawberry.

Then jump up and pick an apple!

Options:

Pick 10 strawberries and 10 apples

Pick 20 strawberries and 20 apples

Pick 30 strawberries and 30 apples

Popcorn!

Bend your knees and crouch
down to the ground.
Then JUMP UP FAST,
just like a corn popping!

(Repeat 5, 10, or 15 times)

Count the number of times you
have "popped."

Pop as many times as you want!

Sway Like a Tree

Pretend you are a tree.
Your arms are your branches.
It is a windy day outside and
your branches are swaying
back and forth.

While your branches are swaying:

1. Practice times tables

2. List your favorite foods

3. Name 5 cities near you

4. Name 5 states near you

Toss The Ball

(You will need a small, soft, squishy ball)

Everyone stand near your desk or in a circle and jump up and down.

The person with the ball will ask a times table question.

They will choose the first person they see raise their hand to answer.

If they are correct,
they toss the ball to that person.

Repeat!

Foot-Alphabet

Stand up straight and tall.

Lift your left foot and use your toes to "draw" the letters of the alphabet, beginning with the letter A.

After completing the alphabet, repeat using the right foot and right toes.

This can also be done with spelling words substituted for the alphabet.

Arm - Alphabet

Stand up straight and tall.

Lift your left arm and use your fingers to "draw" the letters of the alphabet, beginning with the letter A.

After completing the alphabet,
repeat using the right arm
and right hand.

This can also be done with spelling words substituted for the alphabet.

Flap like a bird

Stand up straight and tall and reach your arms up high, then FLAP LIKE A BIRD!

While you are flapping like a bird,

1. Count from 1 to 20

2. Count from 1 to 30

3. Count from 1 to 40

4. Count from 1 to 50

Create your own Activity!

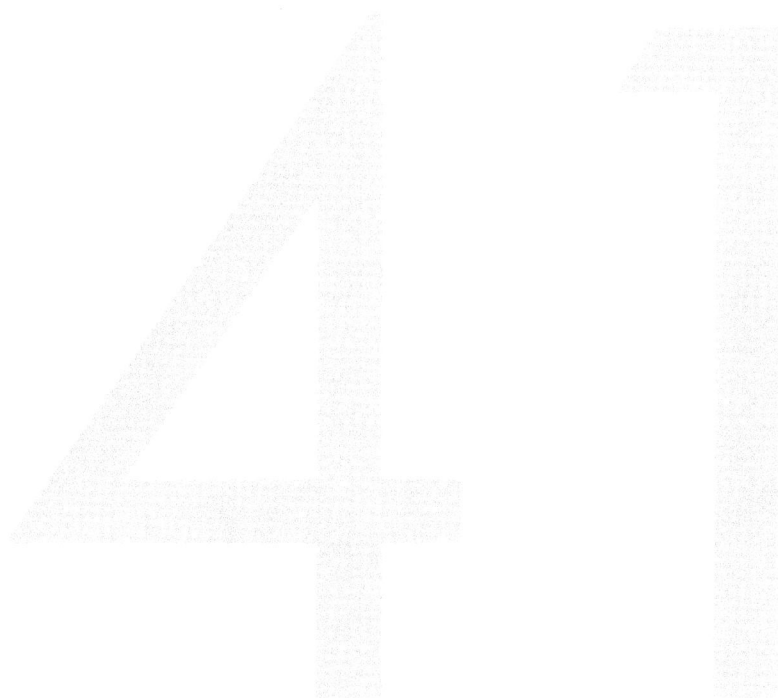

Create your own Activity!

42

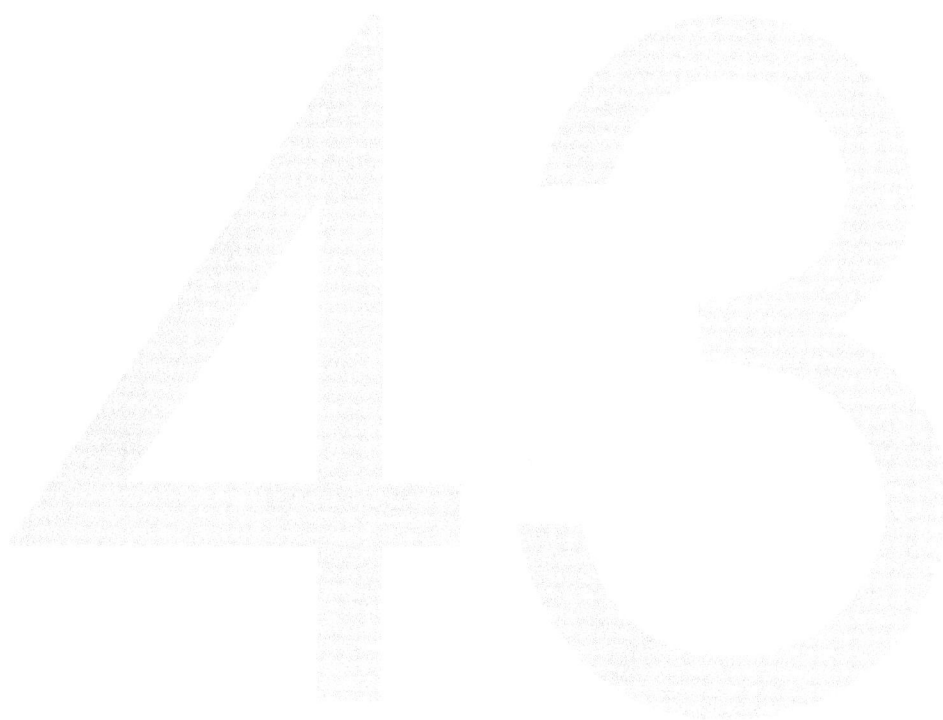

Create your own Activity!

Create your own Activity!